The Wise Woman's Workout

Strengthening Your Body and Mind with Strength Training

By

Maggie Todd

Table of contents

Chapter 1

Introduction: Benefits of Strength Training for Older Women

As women age, their bodies endure multiple changes that might impair their general health and quality of life. One of the most notable changes is the steady loss of muscular mass and strength, a disease known as sarcopenia. Sarcopenia may lead to a decline in functional capacity, which can make it difficult for women to accomplish routine duties and activities. It may also raise the chance of falls and accidents, which can have a big effect on their freedom and mobility.

Thankfully, strength training may assist to counteract sarcopenia and its related hazards. In reality, strength training has been demonstrated to give a broad variety of advantages for older women, both physical and emotional. Let's take a deeper look at some of the primary advantages of strength training for women over 50:

Increased Muscle Mass and Strength

Strength training is one of the most effective techniques to build muscular mass and strength, which may help to reverse the effects of sarcopenia. By partaking in regular strength training activities, women may grow lean muscle mass and enhance their physical endurance. This may lead to enhanced functional capacity and more independence, as well as a decreased chance of falls and fractures.

Increased Bone Density

Bone density gradually diminishes with age, which may raise the risk of osteoporosis and fractures. Nonetheless, strength training has been demonstrated to be an effective strategy to enhance bone density, which may assist to minimize the risk of fractures and other bone-related ailments.

Improved Balance and Coordination

Strength training may also assist to improve balance and coordination, which can minimize the risk of falls and other accidents. By strengthening the muscles that support the joints and increasing general stability, women may boost their overall physical performance and lower their chance of injury.

Improved Metabolism and Weight Management

Strength training may also assist to boost metabolism and support weight control, which can have a favorable influence on general health and well-being. By growing lean muscle mass, women may boost their resting metabolic rate, which can assist to burn more calories and improve overall body composition.

Decreased Risk of Chronic Diseases

Strength training has been demonstrated to help lower the risk of chronic illnesses such as heart disease, diabetes, and arthritis. By increasing general fitness and metabolic health, women may minimize their chance of acquiring chronic disorders and have a better quality of life.

Despite the numerous advantages of strength training for older women, there are still many misunderstandings and myths around this sort of exercise. Some women may feel that strength training would make them bulky or masculine-looking, or that it is harmful or inefficient for older women. Nevertheless, these ideas are not supported by scientific research, and in reality, strength training may be a safe and effective strategy for older women to enhance their physical and mental health.

In the following chapters, we will cover the fundamentals of strength training for older women, including how to get started, selecting the correct equipment and exercises, and building a safe and successful training program. We will also address subjects such as cardiovascular and flexibility training, diet and recuperation, and overcoming typical hurdles to exercise. By the conclusion of this book, you will have all the tools and information you need to begin a successful strength training program and enjoy the numerous advantages it has to offer.

Chapter 2

Getting Started with Strength Training

Strength training is an excellent approach to grow muscle mass, improve bone density, and boost overall physical performance. Yet, for women who are new to strength training, getting started might be scary. In this chapter, we will discuss the fundamentals of strength training for older women, including how to get started, selecting the correct equipment and exercises, and building a safe and successful training program.

Establishing Objectives and Measuring Fitness Level

When starting any training program, it's necessary to establish specific objectives and analyze your existing fitness level. This will allow you to decide the optimum strategy to strength training and guarantee that you are developing safely and successfully. Some frequent exercise objectives for older women may include gaining strength, improving general fitness and mobility, or minimizing the risk of chronic illness.

Selecting the Correct Equipment

Strength training may be done with a variety of equipment, including free weights, weight machines, resistance bands, and bodyweight exercises. The ideal equipment for you will depend on your objectives, fitness level, and personal preferences. Free weights and resistance bands may be wonderful alternatives for beginners, since they allow for a broad variety of workouts and can be readily changed to meet varying degrees of difficulty.

Appropriate Form and Technique

While beginning a strength training program, it's crucial to concentrate on good form and technique to minimize injury and promote optimal muscle activation. This may entail working with a personal trainer or fitness expert to learn the foundations of each exercise and get feedback on your technique.

Beginning with Fundamental Exercises

For novices, it's crucial to start with fundamental exercises that target key muscular groups, such as squats, lunges, push-ups, and rows. These exercises may assist to establish a firm foundation of strength and stability, and can be tweaked as required to suit various fitness levels.

Progressing Safely and Effectively

As you grow more familiar with fundamental exercises, you may progressively increase the weight, repetitions, or sets to continue pushing your muscles and making progress. Nonetheless, it's crucial to move carefully and cautiously to minimize harm and assure continuing improvement. Also, it's crucial to diversify your routines and use a range of activities to reduce boredom and keep enthusiasm.

Combining Cardiovascular and Flexibility Training

Strength training is a vital component of a well-rounded fitness program, but it's also necessary to combine cardiovascular and flexibility training. Cardiovascular activity, such as brisk walking, cycling, or swimming, may assist to enhance heart health and general fitness. Flexibility activities, such as stretching or yoga, may assist to enhance mobility and lower the chance of injury.

Conclusion

Beginning a strength training program may be a terrific approach for older women to enhance their physical and mental health. By establishing clear objectives, selecting the correct equipment and exercises, and advancing safely and efficiently, you may gain strength, improve bone density, and boost overall physical performance. In the following chapter, we will discuss several typical strength training exercises for older women, including how to execute them safely and successfully.

Chapter 3

Building a Strong Foundation

Establishing a good foundation in strength training is vital for women of all ages, but it is especially critical for older women. As we age, we gradually lose muscle mass, which may contribute to diminished mobility, increased risk of falls, and other health concerns. In this chapter, we will cover how to create a solid foundation in strength training, including building excellent habits, concentrating on the core, and moving safely and efficiently.

Building Good Habits Establishing a solid foundation in strength training entails creating excellent habits, such as maintaining appropriate technique, keeping consistent with sessions, and pushing yourself to go beyond your comfort zone. Consistency is crucial, since frequent strength training sessions will aid to grow and maintain muscle mass over time.

Concentrating on the Core The core muscles, comprising the abdominals, back muscles, and hips, are vital for maintaining balance and stability. Concentrating on core exercises may assist to improve posture, minimize the chance of injury, and boost overall physical performance. Examples of core workouts include planks, side planks, and bridges.

Including Compound Exercises Compound exercises include training many muscle groups at once and may be extremely effective for improving strength and muscular growth. Examples of compound exercises are squats, lunges, and deadlifts. These exercises may be done with free weights or weight machines, and can be adapted to suit various fitness levels.

Including Isolation Exercises Isolation exercises concentrate on individual muscle groups and may be beneficial for addressing regions that may be weaker or less developed. Examples of isolated exercises are bicep curls, tricep extensions, and calf raises. These workouts may be done with free weights, weight machines, or resistance bands.

Progressing Safely and Effectively When you create a firm foundation in strength training, it's crucial to advance safely and efficiently. This may mean raising the weight, repetitions, or sets of current workouts, or integrating new exercises into your regimen. Yet, it's crucial to move cautiously and listen to your body to minimize damage and guarantee continuing improvement.

Integrating Recovery and Rest Days Recovery and rest days are vital for creating a firm foundation in strength training. During recuperation intervals, your muscles heal and renew, which may contribute to improved strength and muscular growth over time. Moreover, rest days might assist to minimize burnout and keep motivation.

Conclusion

Establishing a good foundation in strength training is vital for women of all ages, but it is especially critical for older women. By creating excellent habits, concentrating on the core, including compound and isolation exercises, advancing safely and efficiently, and adding recovery and rest days, you may gain strength, improve mobility, and enhance overall physical performance. In the following chapter, we will cover some typical pitfalls to avoid in strength training for women.

Chapter 4

Progressing Your Strength Training Program

When you create a foundation in strength training, it's crucial to upgrade your program to continue seeing gains. In this chapter, we'll discuss several fundamental tactics for developing your strength training routine.

Increase Weight and Volume

One of the easiest methods to advance your strength training program is to increase the weight you're lifting or the volume of your exercises. As you grow stronger, progressively increase the weight you're lifting to push your muscles and continue making progress. You may also boost the volume of your workouts by adding more sets or repetitions, or by including new exercises into your regimen.

Mix Up Your Workout

Mixing up your workouts might assist to push your muscles in different ways and avoid monotony. For example, if you've been performing barbell squats for many months, consider moving to dumbbell lunges or Bulgarian split squats to focus your legs and glutes in a new manner.

Modify Rest Periods

Rest intervals may play a crucial influence in your strength training development. Shortening your rest intervals between sets will assist to boost your heart rate and test your cardiovascular system, while increasing your rest periods can enable you to lift heavier weights with perfect technique.

Integrate Supersets and Dropsets

Supersets entail completing two exercises back-to-back without rest, whereas dropsets require performing an exercise till failure and then immediately dropping the weight and resuming the exercise. Both of these strategies might serve to test your muscles and enhance intensity in your exercises.

Periodize Your Program

Periodization includes organizing your exercises in stages, with each phase focused on various objectives and techniques of training. For example, a strength phase would concentrate on lifting heavy weights with fewer repetitions, whereas a hypertrophy phase might focus on moderate weights with greater reps. Periodizing your program may assist to avoid plateaus and guarantee that you continue making progress over time.

Listen to Your Body

Above all, it's crucial to listen to your body while developing your strength training regimen. If you're feeling exhausted or suffering discomfort, take a step back and review your workout. Pushing through discomfort or tiredness may lead to damage and setbacks, so it's crucial to recognize your body's signals and make changes as required.

Conclusion

Progressing your strength training program involves a combination of challenge and prudence. By progressively increasing weight and volume, mixing up your exercises, tweaking rest times, integrating supersets and dropsets, periodizing your program, and listening to your body, you may continue making progress and attaining your fitness objectives. In the following chapter, we'll cover some tactics for keeping motivated and devoted to your strength training routine.

Chapter 5

Strength Training for Particular Regions

Although strength training gives advantages for the whole body, there may be some areas that you'd prefer to concentrate on more explicitly. In this chapter, we'll study several strength training routines and strategies that may target certain regions of the body.

Arms

For stronger arms, activities like bicep curls, tricep dips, and push-ups might be useful. Adding resistance bands or dumbbells may assist to enhance the challenge and develop muscle.

Core

A strong core is vital for general stability and posture. Exercises like planks, crunches, and

Russian twists may assist to develop the abs, obliques, and lower back muscles.

Legs

For stronger legs, workouts like squats, lunges, and deadlifts might be useful. Changing the style of squat or lunge (such as Bulgarian split squats or side lunges) may target various muscles in the legs and glutes.

Back

A strong back is vital for healthy posture and lowering the chance of injury. Exercises like pull-ups, rows, and lat pulldowns may assist to develop the muscles of the upper and middle back.

Shoulders

Strong shoulders are vital for upper body strength and stability. Exercises like overhead presses, lateral rises, and front raises may target the deltoid muscles of the shoulders.

Chest

For a stronger chest, activities like push-ups, bench press, and chest flys may be useful. Adding resistance bands or dumbbells may assist to enhance the challenge and develop muscle.

Calves

For stronger calves, workouts like calf lifts might be useful. Changing the style of calf raise (such as standing, sitting, or single-leg) may target various muscles in the calves.

It's crucial to note that addressing particular sections of the body should not come at the price of disregarding other areas. A well-rounded strength training program should involve exercises that work the complete body.

Conclusion

Strength training for certain regions may be a wonderful approach to target individual muscles and reach your fitness objectives. By integrating workouts that target the arms, core, legs, back, shoulders, chest, and calves, you may increase strength and muscle in a balanced and efficient method. In the following chapter, we'll cover some advanced strength training approaches for individuals eager to take their exercises to the next level.

Chapter 6

Cardiovascular and Flexibility Training

Although strength training is vital for growing muscle and increasing general health, cardiovascular and flexibility training are equally important components of a well-rounded fitness program. In this chapter, we'll discuss the advantages of cardiovascular and flexibility exercise and present some advice and tactics for integrating them into your workout program.

Cardiovascular Training

Cardiovascular training, often known as aerobic exercise, is any sort of exercise that elevates your heart rate and increases your breathing. This form of exercise may assist to enhance cardiovascular health, boost endurance, and burn calories. Some examples of cardiovascular exercise include:

Running

Running is an excellent kind of cardiovascular exercise that can be done both inside and outdoors. Whether you enjoy jogging on a treadmill or on a path, running may assist to improve cardiovascular health and boost endurance.

Cycling

Cycling is another fantastic kind of cardiovascular exercise that can be done both inside and outdoors. Whether you enjoy riding on a stationary bike or on a road cycle, cycling may assist to enhance cardiovascular health and burn calories.

Swimming

Swimming is a low-impact type of cardiovascular exercise that is mild on the joints. Whether you like swimming laps or joining a water aerobics class, swimming may assist to enhance cardiovascular health and boost endurance.

HIIT

High-intensity interval training (HIIT) is a kind of cardiovascular exercise that comprises brief bursts of intense activity followed by intervals of rest. This sort of exercise may assist to enhance cardiovascular health and burn calories in a shorter length of time than standard steady-state cardio.

Flexibility Training

Flexibility exercise, commonly known as stretching, is vital for maintaining excellent posture, minimizing the risk of injury, and increasing general mobility. Some examples of flexibility exercises include:

Static Stretching

Static stretching includes holding a stretch for a length of time, often 30 seconds to one minute. This form of stretching may assist to increase flexibility and lessen the chance of injury.

Dynamic Stretching

Dynamic stretching includes moving across a range of motion, often in a controlled way. This form of stretching may assist to enhance mobility and prepare the body for physical exercise.

Yoga

Yoga is a method of flexibility training that combines both static and dynamic stretching, as well as breathwork and meditation. Yoga may assist to enhance flexibility, decrease stress, and promote general well-being.

Suggestions for Combining Cardiovascular and Flexibility Training

- ❖ Strive for at least 150 minutes of moderate-intensity cardiovascular activity every week.
- ❖ Integrate both static and dynamic stretching into your training program.
- ❖ Try attending a yoga or Pilates class to increase flexibility and general well-being.
- ❖ Change up your cardiovascular routines to reduce monotony and boost difficulty.

Conclusion

Cardiovascular and flexibility training are vital components of a well-rounded fitness regimen. Combining cardiovascular exercise with flexibility training may assist to enhance cardiovascular health, build endurance, minimize the chance of injury, and improve general mobility. By switching up your workouts and adding a range of activities, you may develop a balanced and successful fitness program. In the following chapter, we'll cover some suggestions and tactics for remaining motivated and conquering typical fitness hurdles.

Chapter 7

Nutrition and Recovery

Strength training is merely one component of a well-rounded fitness regimen. In order to attain best outcomes, it's vital to additionally concentrate on nutrition and recuperation. In this chapter, we'll discuss the significance of nutrition and recuperation in strength training and present some recommendations for improving both parts of your fitness regimen.

Nutrition

Good nutrition is vital for maintaining muscular development, recuperation, and general health. When it comes to strength training, there are a few crucial nutrients to concentrate on:

Protein

Protein is needed for creating and repairing muscle tissue. Strive for at least 1 gram of protein per pound of bodyweight every day, and emphasis on sources such as lean meats, fish, eggs, and plant-based protein sources like beans and lentils.

Carbohydrates

Carbohydrates are the body's principal source of energy. Opt for complex carbs such as whole grains, fruits, and vegetables, and avoid processed and refined carbohydrates.

Healthy Fats

Good fats such as omega-3 fatty acids are vital for decreasing inflammation and promoting general health. Concentrate on sources such as fatty fish, nuts, seeds, and avocado.

Hydration

Hydration is vital for sustaining muscular function and general health. Strive for at least 8 glasses of water each day, and consider consuming a sports drink or electrolyte supplement after extended or hard activities.

Recovery

Recovery is just as crucial as the exercise itself when it comes to strength training. Here are some ideas for maximizing recovery:

Rest

Rest is vital for enabling the body to recover and regenerate muscular tissue. Try for at least 1-2 rest days every week, and listen to your body when it comes to deciding the amount of rest you need.

Sleep

Sleep is vital for helping the body to recuperate and rebuild muscular tissue. Strive for at least 7-8 hours of sleep every night, and consider taking a nap during the day if you feel weary.

Massage

Massage may assist to alleviate muscular tightness and enhance circulation. Try getting a massage or using a foam roller to soothe aching muscles.

Nutrition

Adequate diet is vital for aiding muscle repair. Concentrate on ingesting protein and complex carbs within 30 minutes after finishing an exercise, and consider taking a protein supplement if you fail to fulfill your daily protein requirements.

Conclusion

Nutrition and rehabilitation are vital components of a well-rounded exercise regimen. By concentrating on optimal diet and recovery procedures, you can promote muscle development, minimize the chance of injury, and enhance overall health. Remember to listen to your body and adapt your diet and recuperation practices as required to enhance your results. In the following chapter, we'll cover some suggestions and tactics for remaining motivated and conquering typical fitness hurdles.

Chapter 8

Overcoming Barriers to Exercise

Exercise is vital for preserving physical and mental health, particularly as we age. But, for women past 60, there are distinct challenges that might make it difficult to start and continue an exercise practice. In this chapter, we will examine some of these difficulties and present methods for overcoming them.

Barriers to Exercise

Physical Limitations: As we age, our bodies change, and physical limits may occur. Symptoms may include joint discomfort, muscular weakness, and impaired balance and flexibility, all of which can make exercise difficult and even unpleasant.

Fear of Injury: Many women over 60 may have a fear of harm while exercise, particularly if they have underlying physical restrictions. This dread might make individuals cautious to start exercising or attempt new hobbies.

Lack of Motivation: For some women, particularly those who may have retired or have fewer social contacts, finding desire to exercise might be tough. Without a defined objective or motivation, exercise may seem like a burden.

Lack of Knowledge: Some women over 60 may not know where to start with exercise or what sorts of activities are acceptable for their age and fitness level. This lack of understanding might make individuals afraid to start exercising.

Time Constraints: Many women over 60 may have hectic schedules with family duties or other commitments, making it difficult to find time for exercise.

Suggestions for Overcoming Barriers to Exercise for Women Over 60

Speak with a Doctor: Before beginning any fitness plan, it is necessary to contact with a doctor to confirm that there are no underlying health conditions that may be aggravated by exercise. A doctor may also give recommendations on acceptable forms of exercise and adaptations for existing physical restrictions.

Start Slowly: Beginning with mild, low-impact exercises such as walking, swimming, or yoga may assist ease into a new workout regimen and avoid injury. Gradually increasing the intensity and duration of exercise may help increase strength and endurance over time.

Locate a Workout Buddy: Having a workout companion may give inspiration and accountability for adhering to an exercise plan. Joining a fitness class or organization may also give social ties and a feeling of community.

Establish Reasonable Goals: Having realistic objectives, such as exercising for a set amount of time each week or completing a certain fitness regimen, may give motivation and a feeling of success.

Get Expert Help: Working with a personal trainer or physical therapist may give individualized direction and adaptations for current physical restrictions. They may also assist build a safe and successful fitness regimen.

Integrate Exercise into Everyday Life: Discovering methods to incorporate exercise into daily life, such as taking the stairs instead of the elevator or performing stretches while watching TV, will assist boost total physical activity levels.

Make Exercise Enjoyable: Discovering things that are pleasurable and engaging, such as dancing, gardening, or hiking, may assist enhance motivation and make exercise seem less like a work.

conclusion

Exercise is vital for preserving physical and mental health, particularly as we age. For women over 60, there may be special challenges to establishing and sustaining an exercise practice. Yet, with the correct tactics and support, these obstacles may be overcome, and exercise can become a regular and joyful part of everyday life.

Chapter 9

Conclusion: Summary and Final Thoughts

In this book, we have investigated the advantages of strength training for women and offered practical advice and direction for getting started with a strength training regimen. Here, we will highlight some of the important points and share some last views on strength training for women.

Advantages of Strength Training for Women

Strength training provides a broad variety of advantages for women of all ages, including:

Improved Muscle Strength and Tone: Strength training may help grow and maintain muscular mass, which can contribute to enhanced strength, endurance, and general fitness.

Increased Bone Health: Strength training may help enhance bone density and lower the risk of osteoporosis, particularly in women after menopause.

Improved Metabolism: Developing and maintaining muscle mass may aid enhance metabolism and burn more calories at rest.

Reduced Risk of Injury: Strength training may assist improve balance, stability, and general physical function, lowering the risk of falls and injuries.

Increased Mental Health: Strength training may help decrease stress and anxiety, boost self-confidence, and promote general mental wellness.

Suggestions for Starting Started with Strength Training

If you are new to strength training or have not done it in a while, here are some pointers for getting started:

Start Slowly: Beginning with lesser weights and easier workouts may help develop confidence and avoid injury.

Get Expert Help: Working with a personal trainer or fitness professional may give specific coaching and ensure that you are employing appropriate form and technique.

Consistency is Key: Regularly adding strength training into your fitness regimen may assist optimize the advantages and assure improvement over time.

Change Your Routine: Changing your workouts and utilizing various weights and equipment will help minimize boredom and guarantee that all muscle areas are stimulated.

Listen to Your Body: Pay attention to how your body feels during and after exercise, and make modifications as required to avoid injury and promote optimum improvement.

Final Thoughts

Strength training is a vital component of a well-rounded fitness program for women of all ages. Yoga provides a broad variety of physical and mental health advantages, and with the correct instruction and attitude, it can be safe and pleasant for everyone. Remember to start cautiously, seek expert advice, and listen to your body, and you will be on your path to increasing strength and improving your overall health and wellness.